Cholesterol and Inflammation

A Naturopathic Approach

Jane Semple, MA, ND

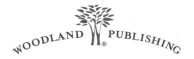

WOODLAND PUBLISHING

For permissions, ordering information or discount pricing, contact Woodland Publishing, 448 East 800 North, Orem, Utah 84097

Visit our Web site: www.woodlandpublishing.com
Toll-free number: (800) 777-2665

The information in this book is for educational purposes only and is not recommended as a means of diagnosing or treating an illness. All matters concerning physical and mental health should be supervised by a health practitioner knowledgeable in treating that particular condition. Neither the publisher nor the author directly or indirectly dispenses medical advice, nor do they prescribe any remedies or assume any responsibility for those who choose to treat themselves.

Cataloging-in-Publication data is available from the Library of Congress.

ISBN 978-1-58054-108-4

Printed in the United States of America

Contents

According to the United States Department of Agriculture (USDA), the economic impact of cardiovascular disease in the United States exceeds $80 billion yearly. Instead of treating cardiovascular disease, conventional medicine identifies a single symptom of the disease, like high cholesterol or high blood pressure, then uses drugs to control the symptom. It's rare to find a case where a single factor is responsible for elevated cholesterol, and cholesterol should not be reduced to a single number for the purpose of treatment.

Cholesterol and related sterols are important to your body for the following reasons:

- All human cells contain cholesterol, which is needed to maintain cell membranes and for cell growth and division.
- Sterols serve as "waterproofing" for the epidermis, the tissue covering the surface of the skin.
- Cholesterol constitutes one half of the dry weight of the cerebral cortex, providing a protective layer for brain cells.
- Sterols are a component of elastin and collagen, the body's connective tissues.
- Cholesterol is needed for the production of the sex hormones estrogen (estradiol, estrone, and estriol), progesterone and testosterone, which help regulate sexual functions.
- The adrenal glands, which sit atop the kidneys, are yellowish in color due to the presence of cholesterol and fatty acids. The adrenal glands contain three distinct zones, all producing different steroid hormones. These hormones regulate such body functions as mineral balance, blood glucose levels, release of amino acids from muscles and lipids from adipose tissue, heart activity, blood pressure and cellular metabolism.
- Calcitonin is a steroid hormone released by the parathyroid glands that's responsible for regulating blood calcium levels.
- Cholesterol is the precursor to vitamin D, which enhances calcium absorption.
- The liver produces bile salt steroids, which interact with fats in the intestinal tract to facilitate the digestion of dietary fats.

Medical investigators at the USDA (U.S. Department of Agriculture) reported that cholesterol plays an important role in protecting against aging of the brain in addition to protecting the heart. The USDA researchers reported that cholesterol serves as an antioxidant in the body, reducing the effects of oxidative stress. (Joseph, 1997)

Cholesterol is obtained from two sources—diet and synthesis within the body. Dietary cholesterol accounts for only about 20 percent of the cholesterol in the bloodstream. The body produces the remainder from saturated fats. If the dietary supply of cholesterol is reduced, the body synthesizes more to maintain acceptable levels in the blood. So, if you are trying to reduce cholesterol levels, you must reduce both cholesterol and saturated fat in your diet.

Lipids are an important energy source; they provide raw materials needed for energy production when glucose supplies are limited. The nervous system (including the brain) requires pure glucose from carbohydrates for its energy needs, while other tissues cycle between lipid and carbohydrate metabolism. Liver cells, cardiac muscle, skeletal muscle fibers and many other cells can utilize lipids for energy production when glucose supplies are limited.

Types of Cholesterol

Cholesterol is a lipoprotein (lipid plus protein). Lipoproteins are classified according to size and relative proportion of lipid versus protein. Although new research that increases our understanding of physiological processes is constantly being done, the following explanation is a simplification that should serve our purposes.

- Triglycerides, the largest and least dense lipoprotein, transfer energy from food into cells. Triglycerides are the main dietary source of fat used for energy production. Excess levels are deposited into fatty tissue.
- Very-low-density lipoprotein (VLDL) consists mainly of triglycerides and small amounts of cholesterol. The primary function of VLDL is to transport triglycerides throughout the body. After VLDL transfers enough triglycerides, it becomes LDL.
- Low-density lipoprotein (LDL) contains more cholesterol and fewer triglycerides. This is the cholesterol delivered for use in the body. LDL cholesterol is considered unhealthy or "bad" cholesterol. Remember that "L" is for lousy.
- High-density lipoprotein (HDL) contains roughly equal amounts of cholesterol and protein. HDL is made in the liver and intestine. The function of HDL is to return unused cholesterol to the liver. HDL is referred to as "good" cholesterol. For tests we remembered "H" is for healthy.

In reading laboratory test results, cholesterol is reported in milligrams per deciliter (mg/dl). For simplification, I will use the cholesterol number and omit mg/dl. For example, instead of 220 mg/dl, I will simply indicate 220.Total cholesterol equals HDL plus VLDL plus LDL. Laboratories usually test total cholesterol, HDL, and triglycerides, and then calculate VLDL and LDL. VLDL is calculated as triglycerides divided by five. LDL is calculated as total cholesterol minus HDL minus VLDL. Total cholesterol should be reasonably stable over the short term (plus or minus 10 percent).

As an example, a laboratory blood test showed that one client's total cholesterol was 248. The client then began a diet and supplement program, and was pleased when a health fair cholesterol screening showed a reduction to 227 only four weeks later. However, another health fair screening showed 237 two weeks after that, which confused her. I explained that the margin for error in such cholesterol tests is plus or minus 10 percent, though 237 is the average of the readings.

Triglycerides vary depending on recent diet, so blood should be drawn after a ten- to twelve-hour fast. One blood type O client (see section on food) didn't follow her prescribed diet and ate excessive wheat in the form of bread the month before her blood test. She then followed the prescribed diet more carefully and had another cholesterol test six months later. Comparison of the two tests: total cholesterol 270 to 241; triglycerides 287 to 197; HDL 56 to 59; LDL 157 to 143; and VLDL 57 to 39. Nearly all of the cholesterol drop was related to a decrease in triglycerides, which was related to a reduction in the consumption of wheat products.

Acceptable Cholesterol Limits

The goal is to keep cholesterol levels within acceptable limits, not to eliminate cholesterol from your bloodstream. The medical textbook *Fundamentals of Anatomy and Physiology,* by Frederic Martini, notes that acceptable cholesterol levels increase with age. Levels are considered unhealthy if they are higher than 185 for a male at age 19, or higher than 250 at age 70. For females, healthy levels are below 190 at age 19, but can increase to 275 at age 70. If the HDL level is below 35 or the total cholesterol-to-HDL ratio is above 4.5, a person may be at risk regardless of the total.

Current Medical Diagnosis and Treatment (CMDT) is considered the standard of care for conventional physicians. According to the 2004 edition, middle-aged men whose total serum cholesterol is above 230 have a risk of coronary death before age 65 of about 10 percent. Men in the lowest quintile, below 170, have about a 3 percent chance. However, it is possible that the real reason for fewer cardiovascular deaths is due to diet and lifestyle changes that are keeping cholesterol levels naturally low, rather than artificially lowering cholesterol with drugs .

Death from coronary heart disease is less common in women before the age of 65, being about one-third the risk of men. The effect of HDL in women is greater (the higher the better), whereas the effects of total and LDL cholesterol are smaller. (CMDT, 2004) Thus, cholesterol screening and treatment in women are questionable. All of these relationships diminish with age for both men and women. The CMDT lists cholesterol as a risk factor only until age 75. After age 75, cholesterol is not a risk factor. In other words, cholesterol is a risk factor for younger individuals, not older individuals. Drug treatment in older adults is controversial.

Studies from Leiden University Medical Center in the Netherlands indicate that in people over age 85, high blood cholesterol levels are associated with longevity and good health, owing to a lower mortality from both cancer and infectious disease. "Our study shows that a high serum blood cholesterol concentration is not a risk factor for cardiovascular disease in people aged 85 years and over—on the contrary, it is associated with longevity." (Weverling-Rijnsburger, 1997)

For younger adults, the optimal level for LDL cholesterol is below 130; 130 to 190 is borderline; anything above 190 is considered high.

Desirable levels for HDL are above 40 for men and above 50 for women, though I have seen variations. HDL above 70 is referred to as "longevity syndrome;" people with high HDL seem to live long lives regardless of total cholesterol levels.

The desirable values for triglyceride levels are usually below 150. However, like cholesterol, healthy values for triglycerides change with age.

Infants	5 to 40
5 to 11 year olds	10 to 130
12 to 29 year olds	10 to 140
30 to 39 year olds	20 to 150
40 to 49 year olds	30 to 160
50 and older	40 to 190

In looking at cholesterol, ratios are more important than raw numbers. A ratio of total cholesterol to HDL cholesterol under 5.5 indicates low risk. A ratio of LDL cholesterol to HDL cholesterol under 3.5 indicates low risk.

Familial hypercholesterolemia (inherited high cholesterol) affects about one in a million people. This is a genetic problem in which LDL receptors are absent or defective on cell surfaces, resulting in unregulated LDL synthesis. People with a single defective gene may have cholesterol levels that are twice as high as normal, putting them at risk for heart disease in their 30s and 40s. People with two abnormal genes have LDL levels up to eight times normal, putting them at risk in childhood. Genetic disorders are beyond the scope of this book. Though diet, lifestyle and supplement recommendations would be helpful, they may not be sufficient.

Cholesterol-lowering Drugs

Drugs called statins reduce cholesterol by interfering with cholesterol production in the liver. These drugs include atorvastatin (Lipitor), cerivastatin (Baycol), lovastatin (Altoprev or Mevacor), pravastatin (Pravachol), simvastatin (Zocor) and rosuvastatin (Crestor). I will refer to this group simply as statins or by brand name, such as Lipitor, rather than the lesser-known generic name, atorvastatin.

Side effects of statin drugs include headache, abdominal pain, constipation, diarrhea, indigestion, flatulence, thrombocytopenia (decrease in platelets, which are important to proper blood clotting), liver dysfunction (including increase in liver enzymes), arthralgia (joint pain) and myalgia (muscle pain).

Statin drugs have been linked to severe muscle deterioration, which does not necessarily resolve when drugs are discontinued. I have two clients who had been on long-term statin drugs and were diagnosed with adult-onset muscular dystrophy. These are women who once enjoyed being active, but now cannot walk without assistance. In addition, though their cholesterol levels increased significantly when they discontinued the drug, neither one has suffered a cardiovascular event.

The drug Baycol was pulled from the market in 2001 after 31 people died from rhabdomyolysis, a type of muscle tissue breakdown that leads to kidney failure. Dr. Sidney Wolfe of the consumer group Public Citizen has been trying to get Crestor pulled from the market as well. Public Citizen notes that Crestor causes kidney problems and muscle weakness two to eight times more frequently than other statin drugs. Because all statin drugs have a similar mechanism of action, and because all statin drugs pose such serious health risks, there is a real need to reexamine the use of this whole class of drugs.

There is another class of cholesterol-lowering drugs called resins or bile acids, which include cholestyramine (Nova-Cholamine and Questran) and colestipol (Colestid). Side effects may include abdominal discomfort, diarrhea, constipation, gastrointestinal (GI) bleeding, fecal impaction, hemorrhoids, anemia (due to bleeding), muscle and joint pain and osteoporosis (likely from reduced vitamin D).

Ezetimibe (Zetia) inhibits cholesterol absorption. Side effects include abdominal pain, diarrhea, muscle and joint pain and increased liver enzymes. I see the use of this drug increasing with the level of advertising. A few of my clients have had such explosive diarrhea that they had to discontinue taking Zetia. There are so many herbs that can absorb cholesterol safely and inexpensively; I cannot imagine why someone would choose to take such an expensive and potentially toxic drug.

Niacin has also been prescribed for lowering cholesterol. High-dose niacin can cause cardiac arrhythmia, atrial fibrillation, excessively low blood pressure, diarrhea, nausea and liver dysfunction.

Another class of drugs that lowers triglyceride levels includes fenobirate (Lofibra or TriCor) and gemfibrozil (Lopid). Side effects include abdominal pain, indigestion, acute appendicitis, pancreatitis, constipation, diarrhea, nausea, bile duct obstruction and increased liver enzymes, as well as decreased white blood cell and platelet counts.

How Good Is Statin Drug Research?

Clearly, the answer is not very good. I did research for 17 years, so I am in a position to comment. One example is a very large study of over 20,000 high-risk individuals. The findings claim that a statin drug reduced all-cause mortality significantly over five years. The coronary death rate was 6.9 percent for the placebo group versus 5.7 percent for the statin group, a reduction of 1.2 percent. In research lingo this is reported as a 21 percent reduction (1.2 divided by 5.7).

By the end of the study, one in six statin group participants had stopped taking their statin drug, while one in three placebo group participants were given a statin drug by their physician. Each person was left in their original group, statin or placebo, whether or not they were taking a statin drug. Thus we are comparing a mixed group to a mixed group. It is interesting to note that during the time they participated in the study, the placebo group was more likely to smoke and to be treated for hypertension, both of which are risk factors for coronary death. So, the 1.2 percent increase in death rate may have been due to smoking or hypertension, not cholesterol.

Lowering Cholesterol May Not Be All It's Cracked Up to Be

The Lipid Research Clinics Primary Prevention and Helsinki Heart Trial reported that although cholesterol-lowering drugs reduced the incidence of cardiovascular events, the drugs did not reduce total mortality. Lipid-lowering drugs in the Coronary Drug Project lowered non-fatal heart attacks, but did not lower total mortality. (Alpert)

Although some studies show that cholesterol-lowering drugs reduce cardiovascular deaths slightly, they increase cancer deaths and suicide. The liver is the body's detoxifier. Reducing liver function would be expected to increase immune-related diseases like cancer. The brain requires cholesterol for proper functioning; thus a reduction in cholesterol may cause depression, resulting in an increase in suicide.

In another study, 11,563 patients with coronary artery disease were followed for 3.3 years. Those with the lowest total cholesterol (below 160) had a 9 percent greater risk of cardiac death and a 227 percent greater risk—yes, more than double— of non-cardiac death. The most frequent cause of non-cardiac death associated with low total cholesterol was cancer. (Behar, 1997)

A study reported in the *Journal of Cardiac Failure* measured cholesterol in 1,134 patients with advanced heart failure. Those in the lowest quintile of total cholesterol (below 150) had lower LDL, HDL and triglycerides. This low-cholesterol group also had the poorest ventricular ejection fraction and cardiac output, with a risk of death 2.1 times greater than those with the highest cholesterol. Thus, cholesterol below 150 was associated with worse outcomes in heart failure patients and impaired survival rates. (Horwich and Hamilton, 2002)

Statin drugs block liver production of cholesterol six steps up the chain, affecting much more than cholesterol. Statins reduce liver production of hormones; coenzyme Q10 (CoQ10), which is needed for proper muscle functioning; and dolichol. Dolichol directs proteins in the cells in response to DNA directives. As a result, statin drugs can lead to "unpredictable chaos on the cellular level." In addition, squalene, the step immediately before cholesterol, has anticancer effects. (Fallon and Enig)

According to a report in the *Annals of Internal Medicine,* damage caused by statin drugs is not always caught by blood tests. Even when blood tests for creatine kinase were normal, biopsies showed distinct muscle abnormalities. In addition, during the study patients were able to identify when they were on a statin drug and when they were receiving a placebo, based on muscle weakness and discomfort. Statin drugs can cause muscle destruction, which is sometimes fatal. (Phillips, 2002)

A study reported in the *Journal of the American Medical Association* followed 10,355 people aged 55 and older. One-half (5,170 people) were given pravastatin (Pravachol). After five years, overall mortality and cardiovascular death rates were similar for both groups. (Furberg, 2002) Thus, these researchers started out to show that statin drugs reduce mortality and found the opposite. In other words, $31 million worth of drugs demonstrated no positive effect ($31 million = 5,170 people x $1,200 per year x 5 years).

Another study reported in the *Journal of the American Medical Association* surprised researchers (but did not surprise me) by showing that there was little or no benefit to giving an increased statin dose to people who recently had a heart attack. Those taking a higher dose of 40 and 80 milligrams per day also had an increased risk of muscle-related complications compared to those taking placebo or 20 milligrams per day. (deLemos, 2004)

In a randomized, controlled trial of 5,804 older patients (aged 70 to 82) a researcher wrote, "one unexpected finding that is likely due to chance was the patients in the pravastatin group experienced a 25 percent higher rate of reported newly diagnosed cancers." (PROSPER) The increased diagnosis of cancer should not have been unexpected, as it has been seen in many other statin trials.

Cholesterol functions as a protective cell layer and constitutes 20 percent of total brain matter. A University of Pittsburgh study reported that patients treated with statin drugs for a mere six months compared poorly with patients on a placebo in solving mazes and on memory tests. (Muldoon, 2002)

Dr. Beatrice Golomb, an associate professor at the University of California, has collected data on 500 people who reported having muscle aches, memory problems and neuropathy (nerve damage) while on statins. Statins were also linked to an increase in blood sugar. "There's a multibillion-dollar industry ensuring that you hear all the good things, but no corresponding interest group ensuring that you hear the other side." (Tuller)

Statins were introduced in 1987. While the incidence of heart attack has declined slightly, an increase in the number of heart failures more than doubled from 1989 to 1997. The heart is a muscle, and thus requires CoQ10 for proper functioning. Remember that statins cause CoQ10 depletion, a problem that will only worsen as recommendations for healthy cholesterol levels go lower and lower.

Guidelines published by a government panel in July 2004 called for aggressive use of statin drugs. Consumer groups complain that the recommendations are tainted by the influence of drug companies that both make statins and finance the research. The panelists failed to list links to statin drug manufacturers. Of the nine panelists, six had received grants or consulting fees from statin drug companies. (Ricks)

Researchers at the Cleveland Clinic found that infusions of synthetic good cholesterol (HDL) reversed plaque buildup by 4.2 percent (yes, that is four point two). This was a 16-month trial, which they called a "huge success" using phrases like "fascinating study" and "tremendous potential." (Nissen, 2003) An example of 4.2 percent would be a cholesterol level of 300 dropping to 288, which you could probably accomplish by eating a handful of Cheerios daily.

I had a 74-year-old male client with a severe calcium buildup in one artery. He was told he was not a good candidate for angioplasty, and probably had a year or two to live. The buildup in his arteries was reduced by 50 percent in four or five months of oral chelation at a cost of about $300—which is truly "huge and fascinating." It has been three years and he continues to enjoy good health with minimal follow-up.

The Inflammation Connection

Inflammation was proposed as the origin of heart disease more than a century ago by German physiologist Rudolph Virchow. More recently, Dr. Kilmer McCully, a Harvard researcher, discovered that homocysteine, an inflammatory marker, caused degeneration of arteries. McCully found that men with high homocysteine levels had three times more heart attacks compared to men with lower homocysteine levels. His research referred to a lack of B vitamins and "protein intoxication." (McCully, 1969)

Dr. McCully tried to have his results published. "I hoped it was significant. I had a big laboratory at Harvard. I assumed it would be welcomed." He was not prepared for the violence of the reaction to his research findings. The drug companies had just spent tens of millions of dollars developing cholesterol-lowering drugs. Now a researcher was saying cholesterol was not the problem. Inflammation was the problem and simple vitamins were the solution. McCully's Harvard lab was taken away at the insistence of drug companies. He continued his research in the basement of a Veterans Administration hospital. Dr. McCully received the Linus Pauling Award for his contribution to medicine in 1999. (Lawrence)

The difference between McCully and many other men and women who were ahead of their time is that Dr. McCully was recognized during his lifetime. Most are ostracized by their colleagues, and spend their entire life fighting against a well-entrenched establishment, only to be recognized for their unique contribution decades after their death. For inflammation, McCully recommends vitamin C and digestive enzymes in addition to B-complex vitamins.

Researchers are rediscovering that it is not LDL itself, but the oxidation of LDL that may be the problem in plaque buildup. Researchers now theorize that heart disease occurs when free radicals combine with LDL cholesterol. Jim Morelli of WebMD explains that oxidized LDL causes damage to the lining of the arteries, which eventually results in the formation of plaque. Oxidized LDL creates foam cells, which are fatty streaks identified as a predictor of cardiovascular disease.

Inflammation that smolders for years inside arteries appears to be a powerful trigger of heart attacks and strokes. According to a study in the *New England Journal of Medicine*, deep inflammation is twice as bad for the heart as cholesterol. Dr. Paul Ridker of Boston's Brigham and Women's

Hospital considers inflammation a central factor in cardiovascular disease. (Ridker, 2002) It is interesting to note that in this study, 77 percent of all cardiovascular events occurred among women with LDL cholesterol below 160, while 46 percent of events occurred among those with LDL below 130. This is another nail in the coffin for using drugs to lower cholesterol in women.

A group of 2,491 men and women with an average age of 72 years were followed for eight years. Elevated homocysteine levels were associated with nearly double the risk of vascular disease. Homocysteine was a slightly better indicator of cardiovascular disease in women than in men. (Vasan, 2003)

Why do we hear so little about homocysteine and so much about cholesterol? Dr. Meir Stampfer of the Harvard School of Public Health pointed out, "there is no commercial interest in studying homocysteine, since the way to reduce it—eating less meat and taking B vitamins—is inexpensive and not patentable. On the other hand, pharmaceutical companies seeking to sell cholesterol-lowering drugs are able to fund numerous studies." (Brody, 2000)

In a trial of 16,176 men and women ages 40 to 67, homocysteine was associated with high cholesterol, smoking, high blood pressure and high heart rate. It was concluded that homocysteine was a major factor associated with cardiovascular risk profile. (Nygard, 1995)

Determining which levels of homocysteine should be considered normal or good is quite controversial. Some medical laboratories list 8 to 20 micromoles per liter of blood as normal. The Physician's Health Study indicated that those with levels of 15 micromoles or higher had three times the rate of heart attacks. The Framingham Heart Study considers levels higher than 9 micromoles to be elevated, placing people at increased risk of heart attack and stroke.

The theory is that inflammation damages artery walls, which in turn causes cholesterol to act as a patch—much like putting a patch on your swimming pool liner to plug a leak. Thus, high cholesterol is the messenger indicating that there is an inflammation problem. Another way to look at it is that inflammation is the problem, while cholesterol is the solution.

The drug companies are scurrying to develop anti-inflammatory drugs that will be expensive and have significant side effects. Unfortunately, this approach will prove to be as misguided as statin drugs.

There are simple, fairly inexpensive solutions to inflammation: B vitamins, vitamin E and essential fatty acids are all anti-inflammatory agents. All of these supplements have a significant positive impact on cardiovascular disease. Given conventional medicine's bias against vitamin therapy, physicians may not advise this simple, inexpensive natural approach.

What You Can Do

Exercise

Even modest increases in exercise can cut inflammation and cholesterol. Exercise can reduce total cholesterol while increasing HDL, thus potentially reducing the risk of cardiovascular events.

Walk, join a spa or join a gym, whatever your preference. I walk with a neighbor. One of us calls the other after work and we walk for 40 to 60 minutes, four or five times per week. One evening last winter it was 15 degrees. When my neighbor's phone rang she looked at the caller ID and said, "It's neighbor Jane." Her husband said, "Boy, she's a hard-core walker." We only lasted for 20 minutes, but the point is we walked!

I tell some of my clients to increase their general activity level. When watching television, walk up and down the stairs during the commercials. If your house is full of clutter, put a few things away during commercials. You are not missing anything except a bunch of drug commercials anyway.

Some clients will claim they cannot exercise because their knees hurt or some other excuse. If a person in a wheelchair can exercise, then someone with a bad knee can exercise. Do chair exercises if you need to. See an exercise physiologist who can set up a program for you.

Diet

We all know that increasing our intake of fiber can reduce cholesterol. Oat fiber has been shown to lower cholesterol, whereas wheat and rice bran have little effect. Oatmeal in the morning is a good way to start the day. Use the kind you have to cook, not the packages with sugar added. Oat-based cold cereal, sprouted bread, and oat bread are also good choices. The best cereal and bread is purchased from a health food store or health food section of your grocery store.

Vegetables and fruits are high in fiber. Be sure you are getting seven servings per day at the very minimum. One-half cup of vegetables is a serving. A small apple is a serving, while most apples today are two servings.

My clients have had the best luck with controlling cholesterol and weight by using the diet plans discussed in the Eat Right for Your Type series of books by Dr. Peter D'Adamo, whose work is based on decades of research into how foods react with blood antigens.

In general, those with blood type A will have a problem when they eat a lot of animal products, especially red meats and cheese. One client, a nurse who was a student of mine, went on the Atkins diet. She lost weight, but her cholesterol and blood pressure rose significantly. The Atkins diet recommends too much meat and cheese for blood type A's, who do best with lots of vegetables, along with some turkey, chicken, and fish.

Those with blood type O and B will find that excessive grains, especially wheat from bread and pasta, will increase triglycerides and LDL cholesterol. Those with blood type O do not do well with dairy either, especially cheese. Those with either blood type do well with a lot of vegetables and moderate servings of meat or fish.

Water

While water is not a major factor in cholesterol, it is a major factor in cardiovascular disease. Chronic dehydration is blamed for damage of the endothelium (artery lining), which leads to inflammation. Dehydration is a factor in strokes, blood pressure and atrial fibrillation.

Several years ago, I was teaching a class and I said that dehydration could cause atrial fibrillation. A man in the class had gone to the ER several months before with atrial fibrillation, which converted to normal sinus rhythm once he was put on IV fluids while waiting for a physician.

In a more recent class, I was relaying this story. A registered nurse in the class often worked in a cardiac unit. The following week she converted five out of seven patients from atrial fibrillation to normal sinus rhythm simply by turning up the IV drip, which rehydrated the patient more quickly.

A general guideline for adequate water intake is six to eight glasses of water per day. This does not include coffee, tea, soda pop or fruit juice—just water.

Major Herbs and Supplements

Conventional medicine isolates a single disease symptom then looks for a single agent to treat that symptom. One example is drugs that reduce high cholesterol levels, a symptom of cardiovascular disease. Nutrition experts know that there is no single nutrient deficiency in disease. The University of California sponsored an International Conference on Nutrition in July 1997. Several research presentations showed that one nutrient alone may be ineffective, even counterproductive. Thus, there is not one single magic bullet.

I do not focus solely on cholesterol, but rather use cholesterol numbers as indicators, along with homocysteine, C-reactive protein (CRP), iridology, personal history and family history of early heart-related death. I do not suggest to my clients that they should maintain total cholesterol at any particular number. I counsel clients on total health.

The following supplements are in the order of my usual recommendations for people with serious cardiovascular disease or a high risk for early cardiovascular disease.

Chelation

Oral chelation supplements are specially formulated to provide high-dose nutrients to clear arteries. I find oral chelation helpful for lowering cholesterol, inflammation and blood pressure. Naturopaths use oral chelation, not invasive IV chelation. IVs are expensive, and, in my opinion, rarely necessary.

Oral chelation starts with low-dose supplements, increasing the dose over several weeks until the maximum dosage is attained. The rule of thumb is to stay at the higher dose one month for every ten years of life. Supplements are increased for one month, then tapered off for one month.

Thus, a 50-year-old person would be on a program for seven months. One month of increasing dosage, five months at maximum dosage, then one month tapering off. A 70-year-old person would be on a program for nine months. Keep in mind that maximum dosages are usually given for adult men. Dosages should be reduced for women based on their height and build, not just total weight.

For serious cases, I recommend that the full program be repeated yearly. For a less serious problem, a three-month program every year may be sufficient.

Your naturopath or herbalist should be able to guide you through a chelation program. If you are on an excessive number of drugs, please work with a knowledgeable practitioner.

B-complex vitamins

A study of 80,000 nurses showed that supplementation with folic acid and vitamins B6 and B12 reduced women's risk of a heart attack by nearly half. (Rimm, 1998) Keep in mind that these three B vitamins reduce homocysteine, an inflammatory marker.

One study followed 10,000 men and women for 19 years. Those taking 300 mg of folic acid had a 20 percent lower risk of stroke and a 13 percent lower risk of cardiovascular disease. Folic acid also slightly lowered blood pressure and cholesterol. (Bazzano, 2002)

Another study linked B vitamins with lower heart risk. Six months of folic acid and vitamins B6 and B12 reduced reblockage by 48 percent after angioplasty (prevented, not delayed). The vitamins decreased the need for repeat angioplasty and coronary bypass procedures by 38 percent. (Schnyder, 2002)

Fiber

Fiber absorbs fat and cholesterol in the digestive tract, keeping it from being reabsorbed into the bloodstream. Fiber also absorbs sugar and starches, helping to regulate blood sugar levels. When cholesterol is only slightly elevated, I suggest psyllium fiber or a psyllium combination supplement along with diet and exercise.

According to a review article in the *American Journal of Gastroenterology,* the American Heart Association diet lowered cholesterol from 3 to 7 percent. Supplements did a much better job. Guar gum lowered cholesterol 8 percent, pectin supplements lowered cholesterol 15 percent and psyllium lowered cholesterol 16 percent. (Anderson, 1986)

Psyllium husks or hulls have been well researched for their cholesterol-lowering effects. As an example, 75 patients were given one teaspoon of psyllium three times per day. After eight weeks, psyllium was found to reduce LDL cholesterol 8.2 percent. (Bell, 1989) This would be a very respectable 12- to 15-point drop for someone with LDL of 150 or 180.

Coenzyme Q10 (CoQ10, Ubiquinone)

Dr. Peter Mitchell was awarded the Nobel Prize in Medicine in 1975 for his work on CoQ10. Statin drugs used to lower cholesterol reduce liver production of CoQ10. Reduced levels of CoQ10 can lead to angina, hypertension, congestive heart failure, poor insulin uptake, gingivitis, weakened immunity and muscle weakness. Thus, statin drugs could be expected to lead to any of these conditions.

Two groups of patients with class III or IV cardiomyopathy were expected to die within two years with conventional therapy alone. Those receiving CoQ10 showed extraordinary clinical improvement, indicating that CoQ10 therapy might extend lives. (Langsjoen, 1985)

Heart tissue levels of CoQ10 of 43 cardiomyopathy patients were biopsied. Deficiencies of this important coenzyme were directly related to severity of disease. The researchers concluded that CoQ10 is an effective treatment for cardiomyopathy. (Folkers, 1985)

CoQ10 (120 mg) was tested on 73 patients, with 71 in a control group. All patients had a recent myocardial infarction. In one year, the total number of cardiac events was 24.6 percent in the CoQ10 group, and 45.0 percent in the control group. Events included non-fatal infarction—13.7 percent in CoQ10 group and 25.3 percent in the control group. About half the patients in each group were also taking a statin drug. Fatigue was reported by 6.8 percent of the CoQ10 group compared to 40.8 percent of the control group. (Singh, 2003)

One article reviewed 30 years of research on the use of CoQ10 in prevention and treatment of cardiovascular disease. CoQ10 has potential for use in prevention and treatment of hypertension, hyperlipidemia, coronary artery disease and heart failure. Levels of CoQ10 decrease during therapy with statin drugs, gemfibrozil and beta blockers. The reviewer suggested further clinical trials, but recommended CoQ10 to patients as an adjunct to conventional treatment. (Sarter, 2002)

When a drug depletes an important nutrient, the drug should be administered with extreme caution and the nutrient should be replenished. I recommend CoQ10 supplementation to all my clients, especially those who insist on taking statin drugs. Animal studies have shown that CoQ10 is safe, with no toxicity, even at extremely high doses. Recommended daily dosage is 30 to 300 mg.

Essential Fatty Acids (EFAs)

Saturated fatty acids are abundant in hard fats and are solid at room temperature. They tend to stick together and cause cell membranes to become hard. A diet high in saturated fatty acids chokes off oxygen from tissues.

Unsaturated fatty acids tend to disperse and are anti-sticky. Essential fatty acids (EFAs) are healing acids. EFAs stimulate metabolism, increase metabolic rate and are used as structural components of cell membranes and active body tissues (in the brain, nerve cells, retinas, adrenals, testes and ovaries). In addition, EFAs are used by enzymes and positively interact with proteins. (Erasmus)

Omega-3 EFAs reduce homocysteine levels. (Olszewski and McCully, 1993) In a study involving over 11,000 people who had suffered prior heart attacks, 1 gram (1,000 mg) of fish oil in capsule form daily reduced their risk of heart-related death by 30 percent. The group was followed for 3.5 years. (Marchioli, 1999)

Omega-3 fatty acids prevent further damage in men who have already had a heart attack, and may also prevent a first heart attack in both men and women. Essential fatty acids may stave off sudden cardiac death in people without signs of cardiovascular disease. (Hu, 2002)

A study reported in the *New England Journal of Medicine* followed healthy men for 17 years. The researchers found that omega-3s reduce risk of sudden death among men without evidence of prior cardiovascular disease. This is particularly important as more than 50 percent of all sudden deaths occur in people with no history of heart disease. (Albert, 2002)

The U. S. Department of Health and Human Services analyzed 39 omega-3 studies. Overall, the evidence shows that the consumption of omega-3 fatty acids (EPA, DHA), fish and fish oil reduce all-cause mortality and various cardiovascular disease outcomes such as heart attacks.

The U. S. Department of Health and Human Services also analyzed 123 studies that looked at the effect of omega-3 fatty acids on risk factors and intermediate markers for cardiovascular disease. Nineteen studies on triglycerides showed that omega-3s reduced triglyceride levels by 10 to 33 percent. The effect was dose dependent and generally consistent. Omega-3s generally raised HDL slightly, while the effect on LDL was slight and mixed, indicating that the major benefit of omega-3 fatty acids is related to something other than cholesterol—perhaps inflammation.

In a systematic review of evidence, the Agency for Healthcare Research and Quality (AHRQ) reported that fish oil reduced heart attacks and other problems related to heart and blood vessel disease. In addition, fish oil reduced the risk of reblockage after angioplasty. Fish oil's effect on cholesterol was mainly in the area of triglycerides.

According to Udo Erasmus in *Fats that Heal, Fats that Kill*, healing omega-3-containing foods (in order best to good) include: flax oil, soybeans, fish, walnuts, seaweed, sunflower seeds, sesame seeds, almonds, borage oil, black currant oil and evening primrose oil. *Note: The last three oils are higher in gamma-linolenic omega-6 oil used by adrenals and gonads.*

Killing oil-containing foods (from worst to bad): shortenings, margarine, refined oils, pork, dairy products, roasted nuts and seeds.

I recommend flaxseed oil or fish oil to raise HDL and as a generally protective supplement for anyone with a personal history of heart disease, cancer or with a strong family history of heart disease or cancer. I have found that omega-3s increase HDL and reduce inflammatory markers like homocysteine.

Garlic (Allium sativum)

By 1996 there were over 1,800 scientific studies showing garlic as beneficial in lowering cholesterol, blood pressure, blood glucose levels and fibrinolytic activity. In addition, garlic is used in cancer prevention, and is an antimicrobial, antifungal and antiprotozoal agent. Published studies show that garlic exerts a positive effect on cholesterol (241), blood pressure (96), blood fibrinolysis, coagulation and flow (69), platelet aggregation (82), atherosclerosis (25) blood glucose (31), and garlic also acts as an anti-inflammatory agent (12). (German Commission E)

A sampling of studies includes seven reporting a significant (16 percent) reduction in LDL. (Koch and Lawson) Forty studies investigated garlic's effect on total cholesterol, and found an average reduction of 11 percent. Triglycerides were measured in 32 of the 40 studies, with an average decrease of 13 percent. Most studies used garlic powder capsules. (Brown; Koch and Lawson)

A four-year clinical trial was conducted on 152 adults with significant plaque buildup and at least one additional cardiovascular risk factor. The garlic group had a 3 percent reduction in plaque compared to a 16 percent increase in plaque buildup in the placebo group. (German Commission E)

A twelve-month, double-blind, placebo-controlled study reported triglyceride, total cholesterol and LDL suppression and an increase in HDL. The dosage used was 3 grams of fish oil and 1,200 mg of garlic powder. (Morcos, 2001)

A four-year clinical trial of garlic found a 9–18 percent reduction in plaque, a 4 percent decrease in LDL, an 8 percent increase in HDL and a 7 percent lowering of blood pressure. Reduction of relative cardiovascular risk for infarction and stroke was greater than 50 percent. (Siegel, 1999)

Some studies have shown small, insignificant effects of garlic. I do not recommend garlic as a sole treatment. During most heart-related consultations, I suggest that clients add more garlic in cooking and include a combination supplement containing garlic.

Red Yeast Rice

Appropriate for those with familial hypercholesterolemia, red yeast rice will reduce cholesterol, but it acts like a statin drug at higher doses.

Red yeast rice is my very last choice. I have a product that recommends a maximum dosage of 1,200 mg two to three times per day. I do not have a single client on a dosage of more than 1,200 mg a day.

One practitioner put her elderly mother on 3,600 mg daily. Her mother's mental performance would decline noticeably when on this maximum dose and revert to normal when off the supplement. I provided her with the same information I provide all my clients over age 65, namely a copy of the CMDT page stating that cholesterol is not a risk factor after age 70, and a copy of a page out of *Genetic Nutritioneering* stating that cholesterol is protective after age 85.

Lowering cholesterol artificially is what many conventional medical doctors do; it should not be the focus of naturopaths.

Other Herbs and Supplements

Most people who are worried about cholesterol are concerned because of its link to heart disease. I have included the following supplements due to their support in preventing heart disease in general, rather than any significant reduction of cholesterol or inflammation.

Cayenne (*Capsicum annuum*) stimulates blood flow and strengthens the heartbeat. (Henry, 1986) Cayenne can be used in cases of insufficient peripheral circulation. (Glatzel, 1967)

Capsicum stimulates blood flow while moderating blood pressure up or down as needed. Capsicum can be used in the prevention of heart attacks and stroke. An extract of capsicum has been used sublingually (under the tongue) in mild to moderate heart attacks. I recommend this to my hardcore herbal clients, who would rather ride out a heart attack than go to an emergency room.

Hawthorn berry (*Crataegus laevigata*) is used for angina and arrhythmias and to improve muscle tone, oxygen uptake and circulation. Hawthorn must be taken regularly for best results and is safe for long-term use.

"Hawthorn has a long history of use, confirmed safety and clinical evidence to support its cardiovascular benefits, especially cardiotonic activity. There is significant evidence to support its use in clinical cardiology and by the general public." (German Commission E)

I sometimes recommend hawthorn alone, especially for those who are averse to taking garlic. However, I usually suggest a hawthorn combination with capsicum and garlic for my cardiac clients.

Vitamin C and Bioflavonoids: A bioflavonoid is a pigment within a plant that acts as an antioxidant and enhances the activity of vitamin C.

A deficiency of vitamin C contributes to roughness of the intima (inner surface) of arteries, an indication of inflammation. Dr. Anthony Verlangieri of Rutgers University demonstrated a deterioration of arteries by withholding vitamin C from rabbits, then returning the arteries to smoothness by supplementing the animals with vitamin C. (1984)

It has been speculated that apo(a), an inflammatory marker, thickens arteries to protect from damage due to vitamin C deficiency (scurvy). From an evolutionary perspective, it is better to die from cardiovascular disease after producing children than to die of scurvy before reproducing. (Erasmus)

Serum antioxidant capacity was compared in nine subjects who drank one glass (300 ml) of red wine, nine subjects who drank one glass of white wine and nine subjects who took 1,000 mg of vitamin C. (Folkers, 1985)

Substance	Percent increase at 1 hour	Percent Increase at 2 hours
White wine	4 percent	7 percent
Red wine	18 percent	11 percent
Vitamin C*	22 percent	29 percent

*1000 mg

Vitamin E includes a group of related compounds, including d-alpha, beta, delta and gamma tocopherols and d-alpha, beta, delta and gamma tocotrienols. The body does not recognize synthetic dl-alpha tocopherol, which is frequently sold as a form of vitamin E at large discount stores, and it may actually do harm at high doses .

If you want to increase your vitamin E intake, do not look to get it through food. Foods high in vitamin E are incredibly high in fat. "For now, if someone wants to take a vitamin E supplement, it has low toxicity and a high potential for benefit," according to Sheah Rarback, assistant professor at the University of Miami Medical School.

In the 1950s, Dr. Evan Shute, MD, a Canadian cardiologist, became the first person to document the cardiovascular benefits of vitamin E. He could not get published in the United States.

A study of U.S. nurses and doctors found a 30 to 40 percent reduction in the incidence of heart disease among those who had the highest level of vitamin E intake over an eight-year period. The benefit was greatest in individuals taking more than 100 IU daily. (Diaz, 1997)

The U.S. Nurses' Health Study found a 34 percent reduction in cardiac mortality, and the U.S. Health Professionals Study found a 39 percent reduction in cardiac mortality in those who took daily vitamin E. The Iowa Women's Health Study and the Cambridge Heart Antioxidant Study found a 47 percent reduction in fatal and nonfatal myocardial infarctions (MI's, or heart attacks) in patients with proven coronary disease taking 400 to 800 IU of vitamin E daily. Dr. David Emmert, who coauthored an article published in the *Archives of Internal Medicine*, recommends 400 IU of vitamin E daily. (Emmert, 1999)

The National Cancer Institute, the American Heart Association, and the United States Department of Agriculture all endorse vitamin E supplementation. (Quillin)

A few recent studies suggest that supplemental vitamin E provides little benefit. Each negative study I have looked at used synthetic vitamin E. I recommend 400 IUs daily of a natural vitamin E (mixed tocopherols and tocotrienols) for those who choose to add this vitamin to their regimen.

L-carnitine is classified as an amino acid, though it is the only amino acid that is not used in building proteins. Instead, it transports fats into the mitochondria, the energy center of the cell. A shortage of carnitine can cause triglycerides to circulate in the blood rather than being used by the cell to produce energy. Supplementing carnitine may reduce triglycerides and restore strength to the muscles, including the heart.

Chickweed (*Stellaria media*) contains saponins that help break up fat and fatty deposits. Chickweed may be an ingredient in cholesterol-lowering herbal combinations. Chickweed also helps reduce inflammation, acts as a blood purifier and relieves constipation.

Guar gum contains mucilage, which is an effective fat-absorbing substance. Guar gum is used to lower cholesterol by reducing LDL and triglycerides. In addition, diabetics use guar gum to regulate blood glucose levels.

Guggul lipid has a history of use in Ayurvedic medicine. Guggul has been found to reduce LDL and triglycerides while increasing HDL. In addition, this supplement has been shown to help prevent thrombosis (excessive blood clotting).

Lecithin is an essential fatty substance composed mostly of the B vitamin choline. Lecithin is a critical component of cell membranes, aiding in the passage of nutrients into the cell. Lecithin acts as a fat emulsifier, breaking down fat and cholesterol and reducing cholesterol's "stickiness." Lecithin may be used alone or in fat-absorbing combinations. Lecithin is usually derived from soy or egg yolks. Other sources include brewer's yeast, legumes, fish, and wheat germ.

Chocolate: Researchers at the University of California found that chocolate has high amounts of phenol, a chemical that reduces oxidation of cholesterol. In addition, chocolate contains a significant amount of antioxidants. The amount of phenols in 1.5 ounces of chocolate is equal to the amount in 5 ounces of red wine.

We are doing a dark chocolate study at my office. We have four women in the chocolate group and no control group. So far we are all pretty healthy.

Examples of Real People

A 56-year-old male with no personal or family history of early heart disease was on 20 mg Lipitor, then one year later was on 1,200 mg of red yeast rice daily maximum. Dosage recommendation for red yeast rice is 3,600 mg daily, so he was on a dose of one-third. Lipitor costs more than $100 a month; red yeast rice is $11 per month. Note that the results are nearly identical. After my client's second set of results, I suggested he cut back or eliminate the red yeast rice as I consider it unnecessary with these test results.

	Lipitor	Red Yeast Rice
Cholesterol	196	192
HDL	57	56
LDL	126	116
Triglycerides	63	100
Total to HDL ratio	3.4	3.4
LDL to HDL ratio	2.2	2.1
Homocysteine	5.3	4.9

Note: A ratio of total cholesterol to HDL below 5.5 is considered desirable; a ratio of LDL to HDL below 3.5 is desirable. Acceptable limits for homocysteine are listed as 3.9 to 14.8.

A 72-year-old woman with elevated cholesterol had a physician who wanted to put her on a statin drug. Keep in mind that cholesterol is not a risk factor after age 75, and 275 at age 70 is considered a healthy level. I recommended four capsules daily (two with lunch and two with dinner) of a combination of guar gum, psyllium, chickweed and lecithin, along with two capsules daily of flaxseed omega-3 oil. Not only did her total cholesterol drop, but her HDL rose to longevity syndrome levels. She was quite happy, but her physician still wanted her on drugs; she switched physicians.

	First Blood Test	One Year Later
Cholesterol	267	227
HDL	51	70
LDL	210	148
Triglycerides	45	45
Total/HDL ratio	5.2	3.2
LDL/HDL ratio	4.1	2.1
C-Reactive Protein	0.9	0.6

Note: Acceptable limits for CRP are listed as 0 to 1.1.

A female in her late 40s with no personal or family history of heart disease came in for a consultation. I took into consideration her medical history, iridology and blood tests. I suggested she follow her blood-type diet, exercise, take a mega-multiple vitamin containing a high dose of B-complex vitamins and omega-3 fatty acids.

Her physician ordered tests (values below) just before her first visit with me and again one year later. Note that her physician did not run any tests for inflammatory markers. The client's cholesterol ratios improved significantly. Unbelievably, her physician considered her first test okay (under 200), but recommend a statin drug based on the next year's numbers.

It takes quite a lot of my time to explain to a client what each of these numbers means. Total cholesterol is only one factor. HDL is a more important indicator for women, and the higher the better. It is very difficult for a client to grasp that her physician does not understand the concept of cholesterol.

I showed these test results to a friend, who specializes in cardiology. She could not believe the physician's interpretation of the cholesterol panel. The client eventually switched physicians.

	First Blood Test	One Year Later
Cholesterol	198	203
HDL	45	55
LDL	135	131
Triglycerides	90	85
Total/HDL ratio	4.4	3.7
LDL/HDL ratio	3.0	2.4

Note: Below 5.5 considered desirable for total to HDL; below 3.5 desirable for LDL to HDL ratio.

A female client in her 40s with a strong family history of early cardiac death (prior to 65) came in for a consultation. Her physician considered these cholesterol numbers to be just fine (below 200). I was unable to convince the client that her HDL should be over 40, that her ratios are poor and that she needs to see a physician who will keep track of inflammatory markers. The client was not interested in nutritional supplements, other than to reduce her menopausal symptoms.

Cholesterol	197
HDL	17
LDL	164
Triglycerides	80
Total/HDL ratio	11.6
LDL to HDL ratio	9.6

Getting Your Own Blood Tests

In most states you don't need a physician to order blood tests. I have found that a person of average intelligence or education can, with explanation, understand their blood work as well as an average physician. If physicians are irritated by this statement, I ask you to reread the section Examples of Real People earlier in the booklet.

You may call a local medical laboratory to see if they require a physician's order. You may also go on the Internet to www.checkmyblood.com. You can order your own tests and have blood drawn at a local lab. The results are mailed directly to you so you can keep track of your own blood profile.

How to Use this Book

If your LDL cholesterol or triglycerides are a little too high or your HDL is a little too low, you should be able to correct them yourself by using suggestions in this book. However, please seek the advice of a trained alternative practitioner if:

- Your LDL or triglyceride levels are extremely high
- Your HDL level is particularly low
- You have additional factors that may contribute to cardiovascular disease such as diabetes or uncontrolled blood pressure
- You have a family history of early cardiac death

How to Locate a Practitioner

Look for a natural health-care practitioner near you. Check your local phone directory under Naturopaths, Herbs, or Alternative medicine. You should expect to pay a fee for their services. If you are unable to locate a qualified professional, you may contact the American Naturopathic Medical Association (ANMA), PO Box 96273, Las Vegas, NV 89193. Or visit their Web site www.anma.com. The ANMA is the oldest and largest naturopathic association and has approximately 4,000 members.

Bibliography

"AHRQ evidence reports confirm that fish oil helps fight heart disease." www.ahrq.gov, April 22, 2004.

Albert, C., H. Campos, M. Stampfer, et al. "Blood levels of long-chain n-3 fatty acids and the risk of sudden death." *New England Journal of Medicine*, vol. 346, April 11, 2002.

Alpert, Joseph, MD. *Cardiology for the Primary Care Physician*. St. Louis: Mosby, 1996.

Anderson, J. and J. Tietyen-Clark. "Dietary fiber: hyperlipidemia, hypertension and coronary heart disease." *American Journal of Gastroenterology* 81:907–19, 1986.

Behar, S., et al. "Low total cholesterol is associated with high total mortality in patients with coronary heart disease." *European Heart Journal*, vol. 18, no. 1, 1997.

Bell, L., H. Hectorne, et al. "Cholesterol-lowering effects of psyllium." *Journal of the American Medical Association*, 261, 1989.

Bazzano. Tulane School of Public Health, *Journal of the American Heart Association*, May 3, 2002.

Barney, Paul, MD. *Doctor's Guide to Natural Medicine*. Orem, UT: Woodland Publishing, 1998.

Bland, Jeffrey, Ph.D. *Genetic Nutritioneering*. Los Angeles: Keats Publishing, 1999.

Blumenthal, Mark. *Clinical Guide to Herbs*. Austin: American Botanical Council, 2003.

Blumenthal, Mark, Alicia Goldberg and Josef Brickmann. Herbal Medicine: Expanded Commission E Monographs. Austin: American Botanical Council, 2000.

Brody, Jane. "Homocysteine raising risk for heart disease." *New York Times* and *Cleveland Plain Dealer*, June 19, 2000.

Brown, D. *Herbal Prescriptions for Better Health*. Rocklin, CA: Prima Publishing, 1996.

"Chocolate may help reduce heart disease." CNN Health Page, September 20, 1996.

D'Adamo, Peter, ND. *Eat Right For Your Type*. New York: Putnam and Sons, 1996.

Dean, Carolyn, MD, ND. *Miracle of Magnesium*. New York: Ballantine Books.

DeLemos, J., M. Blazing, et al. "Early intensive vs delayed conservative simvastatin strategy in patients with acute coronary syndromes." *Journal of American Medical Association*, 292:1307–1316, Sept. 15, 2004.

Diaz, M., B. Frei, et al. "Antioxidants and atherosclerotic heart disease." *New England Journal of Medicine*, no. 337, August 7, 1997.

Emmert, David, et al. "The role of vitamin E in the prevention of heart disease." *Archives of Family Medicine*, 8:537, December 3, 1999.

Erasmus, Udo. *Fats that Heal, Fats that Kill*. Burnaby, BC: Alive Books, 1993.

Fallon, Sally and Mary Enig, Ph.D. "Dangers of Statin Drugs." *Healthkeepers Magazine*, vol. 8, iss. 1, 2006.

Folkers, et al. *Procedures National Academy of Sciences*, 82:901, 1985.

Furberg, C., et al. "Major outcomes of moderately hypercholesterolemic, hypertensive patients randomized to Pravastatin vs. usual care." *Journal of the American Medical Association*, vol. 288, December 18, 2002.

German Federal Institute for Drugs and Medical Devices Commission E, Blumenthal, et al. *Complete German Commission E Monographs.* Austin: American Botanical Council, 1998.

Glatzel, H. "Blood circulation effectiveness of natural products." *Medizinische Clinic*, (published in German), December, 1967.

Goldberg, Burton. *Alternative Medicine Guide to Heart Disease, Stroke and High Blood Pressure.* Tiburon, CA: Future Medicine Publishing, 1998.

Henry, C. and B. Emery. "Effect of spiced food on metabolic rate." *Clinical Nutrition* 40:2, March, 1986.

Herb Allure Resource Kit. Jamestown, NY: Herb Allure, 2004.

Horwich, T., M. Hamilton, W. MacLellan, and G. Fonarow. "Low serum cholesterol is associated with marked increase in mortality in advanced heart failure." *Journal of Cardiac Failure*; volume 8, issue 4, August 2002.

Hu, F., L. Bronner, et al. "Fish and Omega-3 fatty acid intake and risk of coronary heart disease in women." *Journal of the American Medical Association*, 287:1815, April 10, 2002.

Joseph, A. and R. Villalobos. "Cholesterol: a two-edged sword in brain aging." *Free Radical Biology and Medicine*, vol. 22, 1997.

Koch, H. and L. Lawson. *Garlic: The Science and Therapeutic Application.* Williams and Wilkins Publishing Co., 1996.

Langsjoen, P., and S. Vadhanaviki. "Response of patients in class 3 and 4 of cardiomyopathy to therapy with Coenzyme Q10." *Proceedings of the National Academy of Sciences*, 82:4240, 1985.

Lawrence, Felicity. "Doctor's story exposes politics of research, profits." *The Guardian* and *Cleveland Plain Dealer*, May 29, 2000.

Lippicott, Williams and Wilkins. *Physician's Drug Handbook*, 11th Edition. Philadelphia, 2005.

Marchioli. "Dietary supplementation with n-3 fatty acids and vitamin E after myocardial infarction: results of GISSI-Prevention Trial." *Lancet*, 354:447, August 7, 1999.

Martini, Frederic. *Fundamentals of Anatomy and Physiology.* Upper Saddle River, NJ: Prentice Hall, 1995.

McCully, et al. "Vascular pathology of homocysteinemia: implications for the pathogenesis of arteriosclerosis." *American Journal of Pathology*, 56:111, 1969.

Morcos. Herbalgram, 2001.

Morellia, Jim. "Is Vitamin E Good for the Heart?" WebMD Medical News Archive.

Muldoon, M., et al. University of Pittsburgh, *American Journal of Medicine*, May, 2000.

Nissen, Steve, MD. "New drug cuts plaque in arteries, Clinic finds." written by Sarah Treffinger, *Cleveland Plain Dealer*, November 5, 2003.

Nygard, O., and S. Vollset, et al. "Total plasma homocysteine and cardiovascular risk profile." *Journal of the American Medical Association*, vol. 274, November 15, 1995.

Olszewski, McCully. *Coronary Artery Disease*, 1993.

Phillips, P., R. Haas, et al. "Statin-associated myopathy with normal creatine kinase levels." *Annals of Internal Medicine*, vol. 137, 581–585, October 1, 2002.

Quillin, Patrick, Ph.D. *Beating Cancer with Nutrition.* Carlsbad, CA: Nutrition Times Press, 2001.

Ricks, Delthia and Roni Rabin. "Cholesterol panel didn't note ties to drug firms." *Cleveland Plain Dealer*, July 16, 2004.

Ridker P., Brigham and Women's Hospital, *New England Journal of Medicine*, 347:1557, November 14, 2002.

Rimm. Harvard School of Public Health, *Journal of the American Medical Association*, February 1998.

Sarter. *Journal of Cardiovascular Nursing*, July 2002.

Schnyder, G., M. Roffi, et al. "Effect of homocysteine-lowering therapy with folic acid, vitamin B12 and vitamin B6 on clinical outcome after percutaneous coronary intervention." *Journal of the American Medical Association* 288:973, 2002.

Siegel. Herbalgram, 1999.

Singh, R., et al. "Effect of coenzyme Q10 on risk of atherosclerosis in patients with recent myocardial infarction." *Molecular and Cellular Biochemistry*, 246:75, April 2003.

Tierney, McPhee and Papadakis. *Current Medical Diagnosis and Treatment.* New York: McGraw Hill, Medical Publishing Division, 2004.

Tuller, David. "As statin use widens, some worry about side effects." *New York Times, Cleveland Plain Dealer*, July 20, 2004.

Vasan, R., A. Beiser, et al. "Plasma homocysteine and risk of congestive heart failure in adults without prior myocardial infarction." *Journal of the American Medical Association*, 289:1251, 2003.

Verlangieri, A. Rutgers University. *The Riddle of Illness.* Keats, 1984.

Werbach, Melvyn, MD. *Nutritional Influences on Illness.* Tarzana, CA: Third Line Press, 1996.

Weverling-Rijnsburger, A., F. Blauw, et al. "Total cholesterol and risk of mortality on the oldest old." *Lancet*, vol. 350, 1997.

Web Sites

www.ahrg.gov
www.herbalgram.org
www.jama.ama-assn.org
www.medscape.com
www.nejm.org
www.webmd.com

About the Author

Dr. Jane Semple received her master's degree from Case Western Reserve, graduating first in her class in 1984. She completed a dual Doctorate in Naturopathy and Naturopathic Ministry from Trinity College of Natural Health. She has been an herbalist and naturopathic practitioner for twenty years.

Dr. Semple was a professor at Cuyahoga Community College for six years and Baldwin-Wallace College for three years. She developed an Anatomy and Physiology module for Trinity College of Natural Health.

She founded the Alternative Healing Institute to bring training for alternative therapies to individuals and medical professionals. She develops and teaches Continuing Education courses for those in the medical field.

Dr. Semple is an active member of the American Naturopathic Medical Association, the Association of Nutritional Consultants, American Botanical Council and Coalition for Natural Health. She is a Health Freedom advocate.

She has been listed in *Who's Who of American Women* since 1985, and *Who's Who in Medicine and Healthcare* since 2004. She was honored as a Woman of Achievement in Ohio in April 2005.

Other Books by the Author in the Woodland Health Series

Alzheimer Disease: A Naturopathic Approach

Blood Pressure: A Naturopathic Approach

Fertility: A Naturopathic Approach

HPV and Cervical Dysplasia: A Naturopathic Approach

Influenza: Epidemics, Pandemics and the Bird Flu

Parkinson Disease: A Naturopathic Approach